The Ultimate Lean and Green Fish and Salad Diet Plan

50 easy to prepare fish and salad recipes for your lean and green diet to boost energy and stay healthy

Josephine Reed

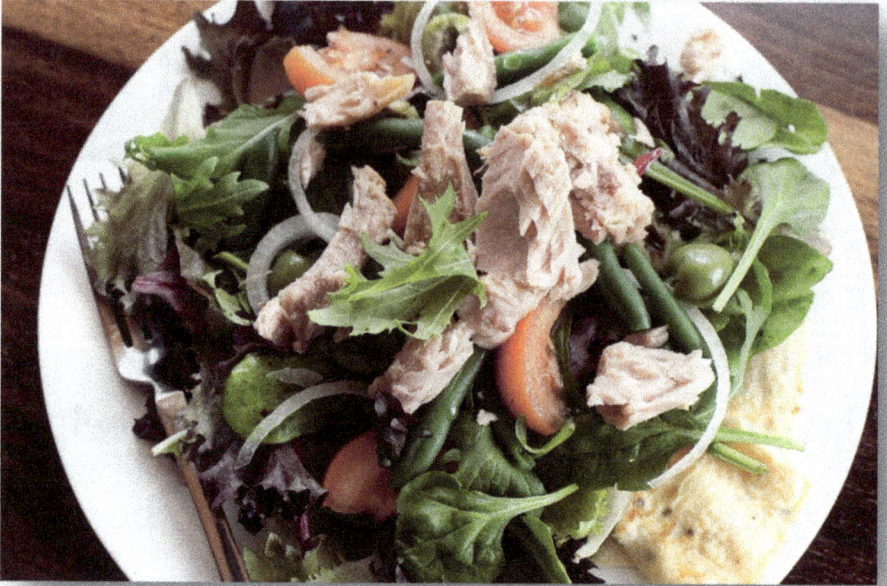

Table of contents

Weight Watchers Macaroni Salad Recipe with Tuna

Prep Time: 15 minutes

Cook Time: 10 minutes

Ingredients:

- 1/2 Cup of Mayonnaise Medium
- 1 tbsp of Red Vinegar
- 1 Tbsp Dijon Mustard
- 1/2 Tbsps Ground Garlic
- 1 Cup of Chopped Celery
- 1/3 Red Onion Cup, Chopped
- 2 Tbsps of Chopped Fresh Parsley
- Salt & Pepper
- 3 Tuna Ounces, In Water
- Macaroni Whole Wheat Elbow (8 Ounces)

Instructions:

1. We must cook the macaroni in salted water first. In order to get the exact times and water measurements, use the kit. Drain the pasta and, after it is cooked, set it aside in a wide tub.

2. When the pasta cooks, the mayonnaise, vinegar, mustard, and garlic powder blend together.

3. Add the mixture of mayonnaise to the cooked pasta, and stir until well mixed.

4. The salmon, celery, cabbage, and parsley are rolled in. Season with salt and pepper to taste.

5. Depending on your tastes, you can serve the dish warm or cold.

Big Mac Salad

Prep Time: 10 minutes

Cook Time: 10 minutes

Ingredients:

Salad Ingredients

- 1 pound lean ground beef
- 1 tsp of Worcestershire sauce
- 1/2 tsp of onion salt
- 1 tsp of minced garlic
- 1 large head romaine, chopped
- 1 large diced tomato
- 1/2 diced small red or white onion
- 1 cup of light cheddar cheese
- 12 diced dill pickles

Dressing Ingredients

- 2 Tbsp of Light Mayo Best Foods or Light Kraft Mayo
- 2 tbsp of nonfat Greek
- 2 tbsp of Ketchup Heinz
- 1/2 tbsp of water
- 1 tbsp of minced white onion

- 1 tsp of sugar
- 1 tsp of sweet pickle relish
- 1 tsp of white vinegar
- dash of salt

Instructions:

1. Spray with non-stick cooking spray on a large skillet. Add the lean ground beef and onion salt and cook, occasionally stirring, for around 5-7 minutes. Using a fork to make the meat crumble.

2. Add sauce from Worcestershire and garlic mined. Stir before the garlic is added. Cook meat until it isn't pink anymore. Take off the heat to cool it down.

3. Measure out 4 ounces of ground beef using a food scale and split equally between the salads. Divide the romaine into four servings, the tomatoes equally.

4. Place 4 ounces of meat on top of lettuce, 1/4 cup cheese, add tomatoes, 2 cups of dressing, and top with diced pickles.

Dressing Ingredients:

1.Whisk or mix light mayonnaise, white vinegar, plain fat or Greek yogurt, sugar ketchup, salt, water, sweet pickle relish, minced white onion, and sugar in a small bowl or in a food processor. Pour into an airtight jar. Place dressing in the refrigerator for a minimum of 30 minutes

Loaded Caesar Salad with Crunchy Chickpeas

Prep Time: 5 minutes

Cook Time: 20 minutes

Serve: 6

Ingredients:

For the chickpeas

- 2 (15-ounce) cans chickpeas, drained and rinsed
- 2 tablespoons extra-virgin olive oil
- 1 teaspoon kosher salt
- 1 teaspoon garlic powder
- 1 teaspoon onion powder
- 1 teaspoon dried oregano

For the dressing

- ½ cup mayonnaise
- 2 tablespoons grated Parmesan cheese
- 2 tablespoons freshly squeezed lemon juice
- 1 clove garlic, peeled and smashed
- 1 teaspoon Dijon mustard
- ½ tablespoon Worcestershire sauce
- ½ tablespoon anchovy paste

For the salad

- 3 heads romaine lettuce, cut into bite-size pieces

Instructions:

To make the chickpeas:

1. Preheat the oven to 450°F. Line a baking sheet with parchment paper.

2. Add the chickpeas, oil, salt, garlic powder, onion powder, and oregano in a small container. Scatter the coated chickpeas on the prepared baking sheet.

3. Roast for about 20 minutes, tossing occasionally, until the chickpeas are golden and have a bit of crunch.

To make the dressing:

1. In a small bowl, whisk the mayonnaise, Parmesan, lemon juice, garlic, mustard, Worcestershire sauce, and anchovy paste until combined.

To make the salad:

1. In a large container combine the lettuce and dressing. Toss to coat. Top with the roasted chickpeas and serve.

Cooking Tip: Don't wash out that bowl you used for the chickpeas — the remaining oil adds a great punch of flavor to blanched green beans or another simply cooked vegetable.

Nutrition: Calories: 367, Total fat: 22 g, Total carbs: 35 g, Cholesterol: 9 mg, Fiber: 13 g, Protein: 12 g, Sodium: 407 mg

Shrimp Cobb Salad

Prep Time: 25 minutes

Cook Time: 10 minutes

Serve: 2

Ingredients:

- 4 slices center-cut bacon
- 1 lb. large shrimp, peeled and deveined
- 1/2 teaspoon ground paprika
- 1/4 teaspoon ground black pepper
- 1/4 teaspoon salt, divided
- 2 1/2 tablespoons fresh lemon juice
- 1 1/2 tablespoons extra-virgin olive oil
- 1/2 teaspoon whole grain Dijon mustard
- 1 (10 oz.) package romaine lettuce hearts, chopped
- 2 cups cherry tomatoes, quartered
- 1 ripe avocado, cut into wedges
- 1 cup shredded carrots

Instructions:

1. Cook the bacon for 4 minutes on each side in a large skillet over medium heat till crispy.

2. Take away from the skillet and place on paper towels; let cool for 5 minutes. Break the bacon into bits. Throw out most of the bacon fat, leaving behind only 1 tablespoon in the skillet.

3. Bring the skillet back to medium-high heat. Add black pepper and paprika to the shrimp for seasoning.

4. Cook the shrimp around 2 minutes each side until it is opaque.

5. Sprinkle with 1/8 teaspoon of salt for seasoning.

6. Combine the remaining 1/8 teaspoon of salt, mustard, olive oil and lemon juice together in a small bowl. Stir in the romaine hearts.

7. On each serving plate, place on 1 and 1/2 cups of romaine lettuce. Add on top the same amounts of avocado, carrots, tomatoes, shrimp and bacon.

Nutrition: Calories: 528, Total Carbohydrate: 22.7 g, Cholesterol: 365 mg, Total Fat: 28.7 g, Protein: 48.9 g, Sodium: 1166 mg

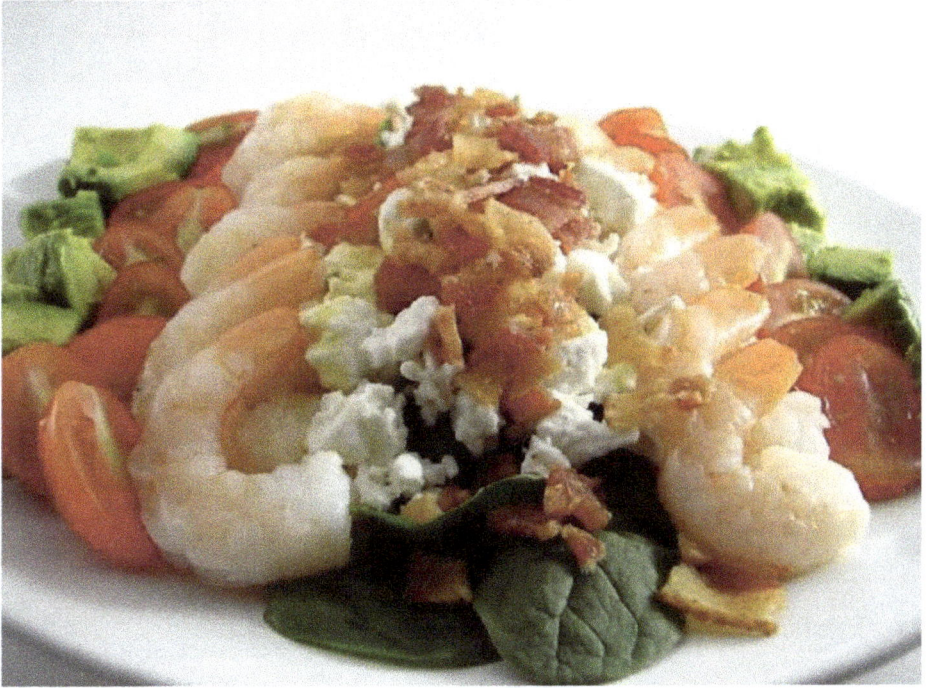

Fruit Salad

Prep Time: 15 minutes

Serve: 4

Ingredients:

For Salad

- 4 cups fresh baby arugula
- 1 cup fresh strawberries, hulled and sliced
- 2 oranges, peeled and segmented

For Dressing

- 2 tablespoons fresh lemon juice
- 2-3 drops liquid stevia
- 2 teaspoons extra-virgin olive oil
- Salt and ground black pepper, as required

Instructions:

1.For Salad: in a salad bowl, place all ingredients and mix.

2.For Dressing: place all ingredients in another bowl and beat until well combined.

3.Place dressing on top of salad and toss to coat well.

Strawberry, Orange & Rocket Salad

Prep Time: 15 minutes

Serve: 4

Ingredients:

For Salad:

- 6 cups fresh rocket
- 1½ cups fresh strawberries, hulled and sliced 2 oranges, peeled and segmented

For Dressing:

- 2 tablespoons fresh lemon juice
- 1 tablespoon raw honey
- 2 teaspoons extra-virgin olive oil
- 1 teaspoon Dijon mustard
- Salt and ground black pepper, as required

Instructions:

1.For Salad: in a salad bowl, place all ingredients and mix.

2.For Dressing: place all ingredients in another bowl and beat until well combined.

3.Place dressing on top of salad and toss to coat well.

Wasabi Tuna Asian Salad

Prep Time: 30 minutes

Cook Time: 10 minutes

Serve: 1

Ingredients:

- Lime juice (1 teaspoon)
- Non-stick cooking spray
- Pepper/dash of salt
- Wasabi paste (1 teaspoon)
- Olive oil (2 teaspoons)
- Chopped or shredded cucumbers (1/2 cup)
- Bok Choy stalks (1 cup)
- Raw tuna steak (8 oz.)

Instructions:

1.Fish: preheat your skillet to medium heat. Mix your wasabi and lime juice; coat the tuna steaks.

2.Use a non-stick cooking spray on your skillet for 10 seconds.

3.Put your tuna steaks on the skillet and cook over medium heat until you get the desired doneness.

4.Salad: Slice the cucumber into match-stick tiny sizes. Cut the bok Choy into minute pieces. Toss gently with pepper, salt, and olive oil if you want.

Nutrition: Protein: 61g, Fiber: 1g, Cholesterol: 115mg, Saturated fats: 2g, Calories: 380

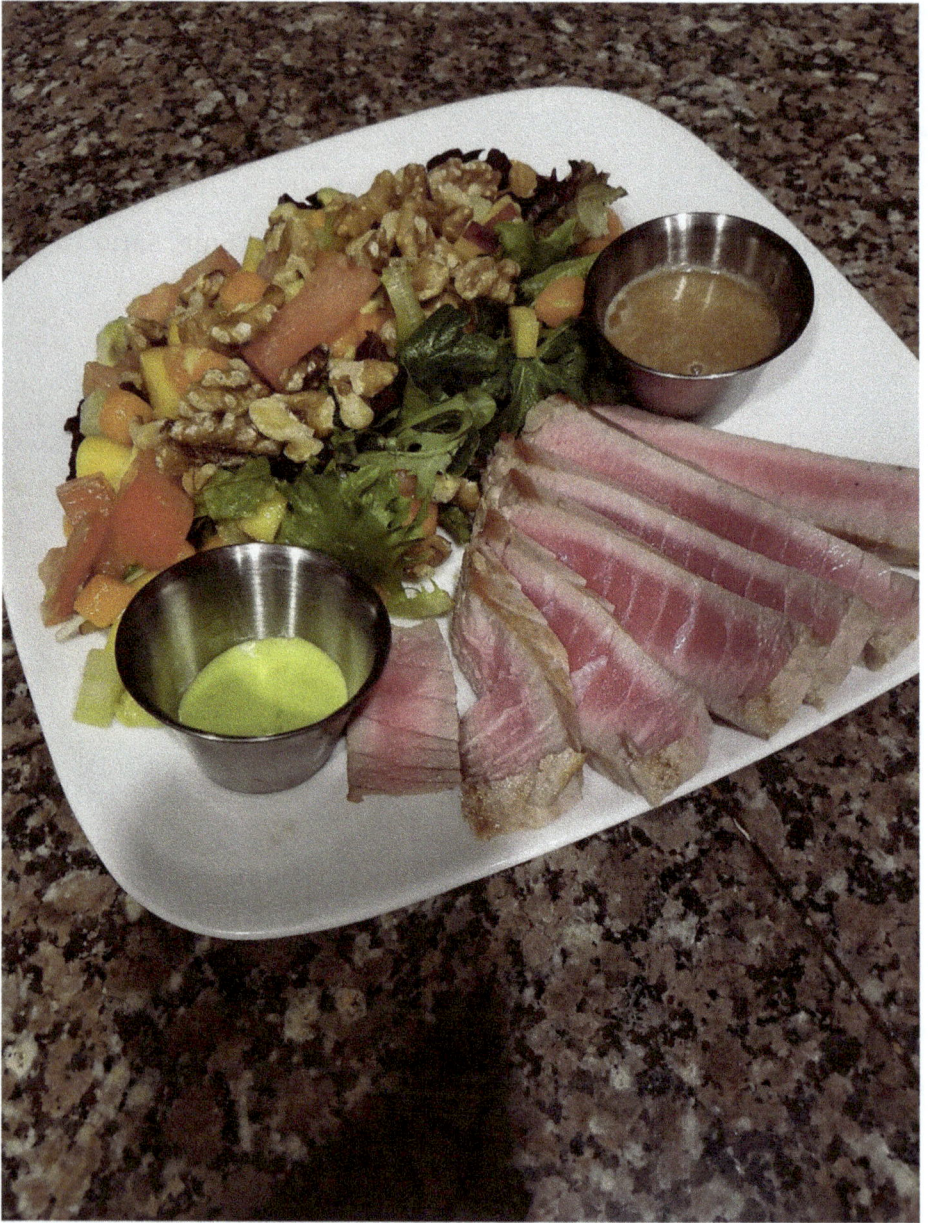

Lemon Greek Salad

Prep Time: 25 minutes

Cook Time: 25 minutes

Serve: 1

Ingredients:

- Chicken breast (140 oz)
- Chopped cucumber (1 cup)
- Chopped orange/red bell pepper (1 cup)
- Wedged/sliced/chopped tomatoes (1 cup)
- Chopped olives (1/4 cup)
- Fresh parsley (2 tablespoons), finely chopped.
- Finely chopped red onion (2 tablespoons)
- Lemon juice (5 teaspoons)
- Olive oil (1 teaspoon)
- Minced garlic (1 clove)

Instructions:

1.Preheat your grill to medium heat.

2.Grill the chicken and cook on each side until it is no longer pink or for 5 minutes.

3.Cut the chicken into tiny pieces. In your serving bowl, mix garlic, olives, and parsley. Whisk in olive oil (1 teaspoon) and lemon juice (4 teaspoons). Add onion, tomatoes, bell pepper, and cucumber.

4.Toss gently. Coat the ingredients with dressing. Add another teaspoon of lemon juice to taste. Divide the salad into two servings and put 6oz chicken on top of each salad.

Nutrition: Protein: 56g, Fiber: 4g, Total carbs: 14g, Sodium: 280mg, Cholesterol: 145mg, Saturated fat: 2.5g, Total fat: 12g, Calories: 380

Broccoli Salad

Prep Time: 5 minutes

Cook Time: 25 minutes

Serve: 1

Ingredients:

- 1/3 tablespoons sherry vinegar
- 1/24 cup olive oil
- 1/3 teaspoons fresh thyme, chopped
- 1/6 teaspoon Dijon mustard
- 1/6 teaspoon honey
- Salt to taste
- 1 1/3 cups broccoli florets
- 1/3 red onions
- 1/12 cup parmesan cheese shaved
- 1/24 cup pecans

Instructions:

1.Mix the sherry vinegar, olive oil, thyme, mustard, honey, and salt in a bowl.

2.In a serving bowl, blend the broccoli florets and onions.

3.Drizzle the dressing on top.

4.Sprinkle with the pecans and parmesan cheese before serving.

Nutrition: Calories: 199, Fat: 17.4g, Saturated fat: 2.9g, Carbohydrates: 7.5g, Fiber: 2.8g, Protein: 5.2g

Potato Carrot Salad

Prep Time: 15 minutes

Cook Time: 10 minutes

Serve: 1

Ingredients:

Water

- 1 potato, sliced into cubes
- 1/2 carrots, cut into cubes
- 1/6 tablespoon milk
- 1/6 tablespoon Dijon mustard
- 1/24 cup mayonnaise

Pepper to taste

- 1/3 teaspoons fresh thyme, chopped
- 1/6 stalk celery, chopped
- 1/6 scallions, chopped
- 1/6 slice turkey bacon, cooked crispy and crumbled

Instructions:

1.Fill your pot with water.

2.Place it over medium-high heat.

3.Boil the potatoes and carrots for 10 to 12 minutes or until tender.

4.Drain and let cool.

5.In a bowl, mix the milk, mustard, mayonnaise, pepper, and thyme.

6.Stir in the potatoes, carrots, and celery.

7.Coat evenly with the sauce.

8.Cover and refrigerate for 4 hours.

9.Top with the scallions and turkey bacon bits before serving.

Nutrition: Calories: 106, Fat: 5.3g, Saturated fat: 1g, Carbohydrates: 12.6g, Fiber: 1.8g, Protein: 2g

Marinated Veggie Salad

Prep Time: 4 hours and 30 minutes

Cook Time: 3 minutes

Serve: 1

Ingredients:

- 1 zucchini, sliced
- 4 tomatoes, sliced into wedges
- ¼ cup red onion, sliced thinly
- 1 green bell pepper, sliced
- 2 tablespoons fresh parsley, chopped
- 2 tablespoons red-wine vinegar
- 2 tablespoons olive oil
- 1 clove garlic, minced
- 1 teaspoon dried basil
- 2 tablespoons water
- Pine nuts, toasted and chopped

Instructions:

1.In a bowl, combine the zucchini, tomatoes, red onion, green bell pepper, and parsley.

2.Pour the vinegar and oil into a glass jar with a lid.

3.Add the garlic, basil, and water.

4.Seal the jar and stir well to combine.

5.Pour the dressing into the vegetable mixture.

6.Cover the bowl.

7.Marinate in the refrigerator for 4 hours.

8.Garnish with the pine nuts before serving.

Nutrition: Calories: 65, Fat: 4.7g, Saturated fat: 0.7g, Carbohydrates: 5.3g, Fiber: 1.2g, Protein: 0.9g

Mediterranean Salad

Prep Time: 20 minutes

Cook Time: 5 minutes

Serve: 1

Ingredients:

- 1 teaspoon balsamic vinegar
- 1/2 tablespoon basil pesto
- 1/2 cup lettuce
- 1/8 cup broccoli florets, chopped
- 1/8 cup zucchini, chopped
- 1/8 cup tomato, chopped
- 1/8 cup yellow bell pepper, chopped
- 1/2 tablespoons feta cheese, crumbled

Instructions:

1.Arrange the lettuce on a serving platter.

2.Top with the broccoli, zucchini, tomato, and bell pepper.

3.In a bowl, mix the vinegar and pesto.

4.Drizzle the dressing on top.

5.Sprinkle the feta cheese.

Nutrition: Calories: 100, Fat: 6g, Saturated fat: 1g, Carbohydrates: 7g, Protein: 4g

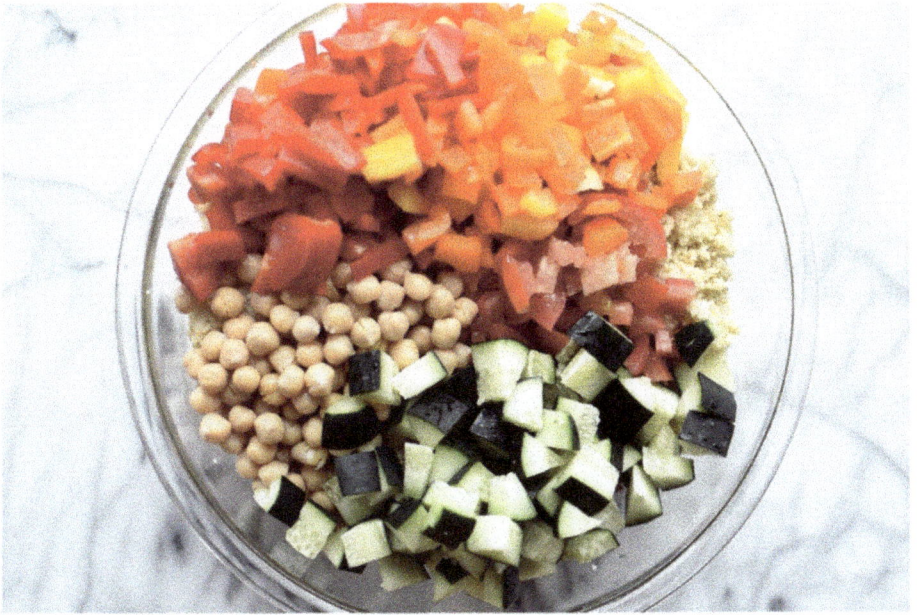

Potato Tuna Salad

Prep Time: 4 hours and 20 minutes

Cook Time: 10 minutes

Serve: 1

Ingredients:

- 1 potato, peeled and sliced into cubes
- 1/12 cup plain yogurt
- 1/12 cup mayonnaise
- 1/6 clove garlic, crushed and minced
- 1/6 tablespoon almond milk
- 1/6 tablespoon fresh dill, chopped
- ½ teaspoon lemon zest
- Salt to taste
- 1 cup cucumber, chopped
- ¼ cup scallions, chopped
- ¼ cup radishes, chopped
- (9 oz) canned tuna flakes
- 1/2 hard-boiled eggs, chopped
- 1 cups lettuce, chopped

Instructions:

1.Fill your pot with water.

2.Add the potatoes and boil.

3.Cook for 15 minutes or till slightly tender.

4.Drain and let cool.

5.In a bowl, mix the yogurt, mayo, garlic, almond milk, fresh dill, lemon zest, and salt.

6.Stir in the potatoes, tuna flakes, and eggs.

7.Mix well.

8.Chill in the refrigerator for 4 hours.

9.Stir in the shredded lettuce before serving.

Nutrition: Calories: 243, Fat: 9.9g, Saturated fat: 2g, Carbohydrates: 22.2g, Fiber: 4.6g, Protein: 17.5g

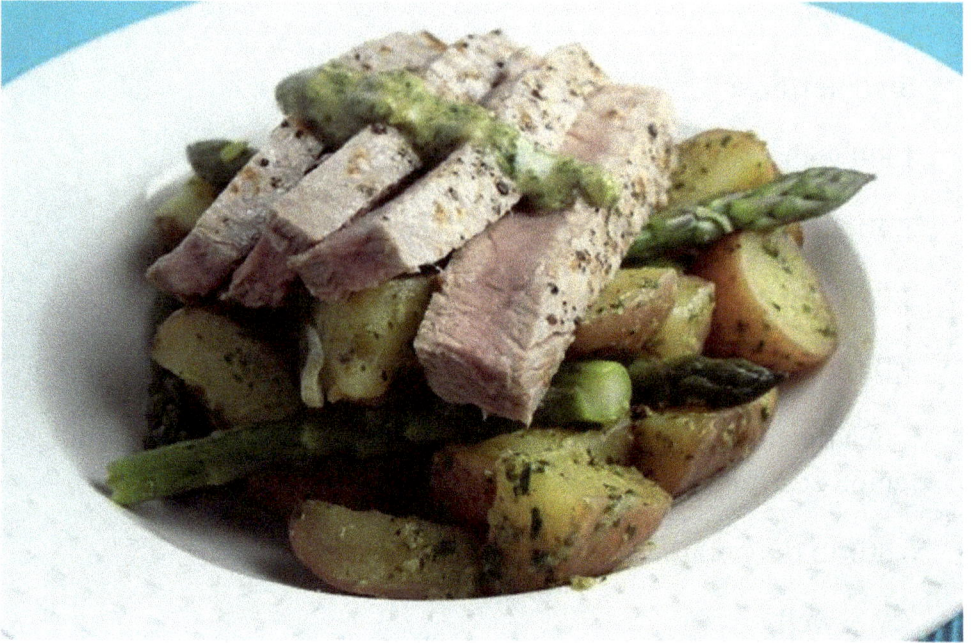

High Protein Salad

Prep Time: 5 minutes

Cook Time: 5 minutes

Serve: 1

Ingredients:

Salad:

- 1(15 oz) can green kidney beans
- 1/4 tablespoon capers
- 1/4 handfuls arugula
- 1(15 oz) can lentils

Dressing:

- 1/1 tablespoon caper brine
- 1/1 tablespoon tamari
- 1/1 tablespoon balsamic vinegar
- 2/2 tablespoon peanut butter
- 2/2 tablespoon hot sauce
- 2/1 tablespoon tahini

Instructions:

For the dressing:

1.In a bowl, stir all the ingredients until they come together to form a smooth dressing.

For the salad:

2.Mix the beans, arugula, capers, and lentils. Top with the dressing and serve.

Nutrition: Calories: 205, Fat: 2g, Protein: 13g, Carbs: 31g, Fiber: 17g

Rice and Veggie Bowl

Prep Time: 5 minutes

Cook Time: 15 minutes

Serve: 1

Ingredients:

- 1/3 tablespoon coconut oil
- 1/2 teaspoon ground cumin
- 1/2 teaspoon ground turmeric
- 1/3 teaspoon chili powder
- 1 red bell pepper, chopped
- 1/2 tablespoon tomato paste
- 1 bunch of broccoli, cut into bite-sized-florets with short stems 1/2 teaspoon salt, to taste
- 1 large red onion, sliced
- 1/2 garlic cloves, minced
- 1/2 head of cauliflower, sliced into bite-sized florets 1/2 cups cooked rice
- Newly ground black pepper to taste

Instructions:

1.Start with warming up the coconut oil over medium-high heat.

2.Stir in the turmeric, cumin, chili powder, salt, and tomato paste.

3.Cook the content for 1 minute. Stir repeatedly until the spices are fragrant.

4.Add the garlic and onion. Fry for 2,5 to 3,3 minutes until the onions are softened.

5.Add the broccoli, cauliflower, and bell pepper. Cover, then cook for 3 to 4 minutes and stir occasionally.

6.Add the cooked rice. Stir so it will combine well with the vegetables. Cook for 2 to 3 minutes. Stir until the rice is warm.

7.Check the seasoning and change to taste if desired.

8.Lessen the heat and cook on low for 2 to 3 more minutes so the flavors will meld.

9.Serve with freshly ground black pepper.

Nutrition: Calories: 260, Fat: 9g, Protein: 9g, Carbs: 36g, Fiber: 5g

Squash Black Bean Bowl

Prep Time: 5 minutes

Cook Time: 30 minutes

Serve: 1

Ingredients:

- 1 large spaghetti squash, halved,
- 1/3 cup water (or 2 tablespoon olive oil, rubbed on the inside of squash)

Black bean filling:

- 1/2 (15 oz) can of black beans, emptied and rinsed 1/2 cup fire-roasted corn (or frozen sweet corn) 1/2 cup thinly sliced red cabbage
- 1/2 tablespoon chopped green onion, green and white parts ¼ cup chopped fresh coriander
- ½ lime, juiced or to taste
- Pepper and salt, to taste

Avocado mash:

- One ripe avocado, mashed
- ½ lime, juiced or to taste
- ¼ teaspoon cumin

- Pepper and pinch of sea salt

Instructions:

1.Preheat the oven to 400°F.

2.Chop the squash in part and scoop out the seeds with a spoon, like a pumpkin.

3.Fill the roasting pan with 1/3 cup of water. Lay the squash, cut side down, in the pan. Bake for 30 minutes until soft and tender.

4.While this is baking, mix all the ingredients for the black bean filling in a medium-sized bowl.

5.In a small dish, crush the avocado and blend in the avocado mash ingredients.

6.Eliminate the squash from the oven and let it cool for 5 minutes. Scrape the squash with a fork so that it looks like spaghetti noodles. Then, fill it with black bean filling and top with avocado mash.

Nutrition: Calories: 85, Fat: 0.5g, Protein: 4g, Carbs: 6g, Fiber: 4g

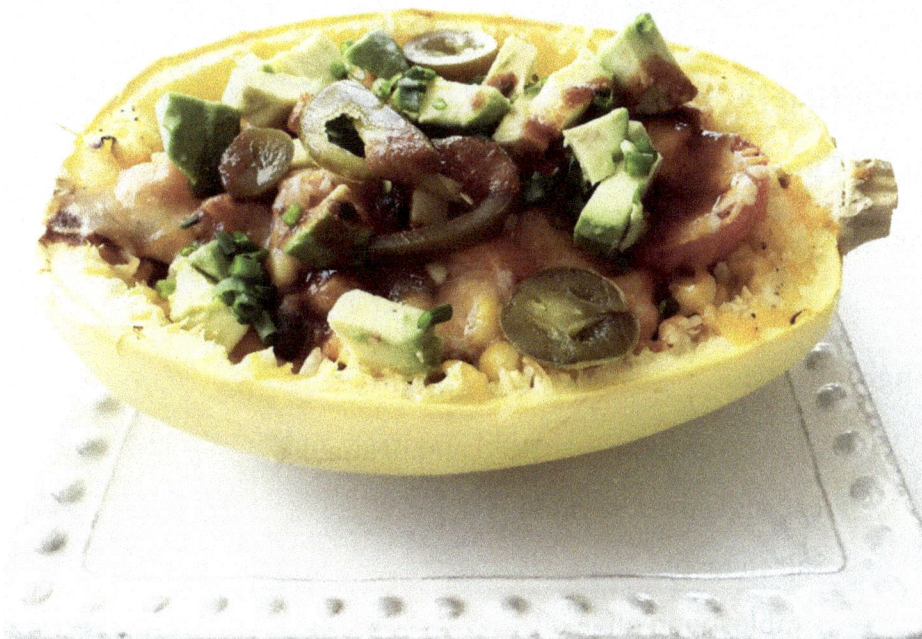

Pea Salad

Prep Time: 40 minutes

Cook Time: 0 minutes

Serve: 1

Ingredients:

- 1/2 cup chickpeas, rinsed and drained
- 1/2 cups peas, divided
- Salt to taste
- 1 tablespoon olive oil
- ½ cup buttermilk
- Pepper to taste
- 2 cups pea greens
- 1/2 carrots shaved
- 1/4 cup snow peas, trimmed

Instructions:

1.Add the chickpeas and half of the peas to your food processor.

2.Season with salt.

3.Pulse until smooth. Set aside.

4.In a bowl, toss the remaining peas in oil, milk, salt, and pepper.

5.Transfer the mixture to your food processor.

6.Process until pureed.

7.Transfer this mixture to a bowl.

8.Arrange the pea greens on a serving plate.

9.Top with the shaved carrots and snow peas.

10.Stir in the pea and milk dressing.

11.Serve with the reserved chickpea hummus.

Nutrition: Calories: 214, Fat: 8.6g, Saturated fat: 1.5g, Carbohydrates: 27.3g, Fiber: 8.4g, Protein: 8g

Snap Pea Salad

Prep Time: 1 hour

Cook Time: 0 minutes

Serve: 1

Ingredients:

- 1/2 tablespoons mayonnaise
- ¾ teaspoon celery seed
- ¼ cup cider vinegar
- 1/2 teaspoon yellow mustard
- 1/2 tablespoon sugar
- Salt and pepper to taste
- 1 oz. radishes, sliced thinly
- 2 oz. sugar snap peas, sliced thinly

Instructions:

1.In a bowl, combine the mayonnaise, celery seeds, vinegar, mustard, sugar, salt, and pepper.

2.Stir in the radishes and snap peas.

3.Refrigerate for 30 minutes.

Nutrition: Calories: 69, Fat: 3.7g, Saturated fat: 0.6g, Carbohydrates: 7.1g, Fiber: 1.8g, Protein: 2g

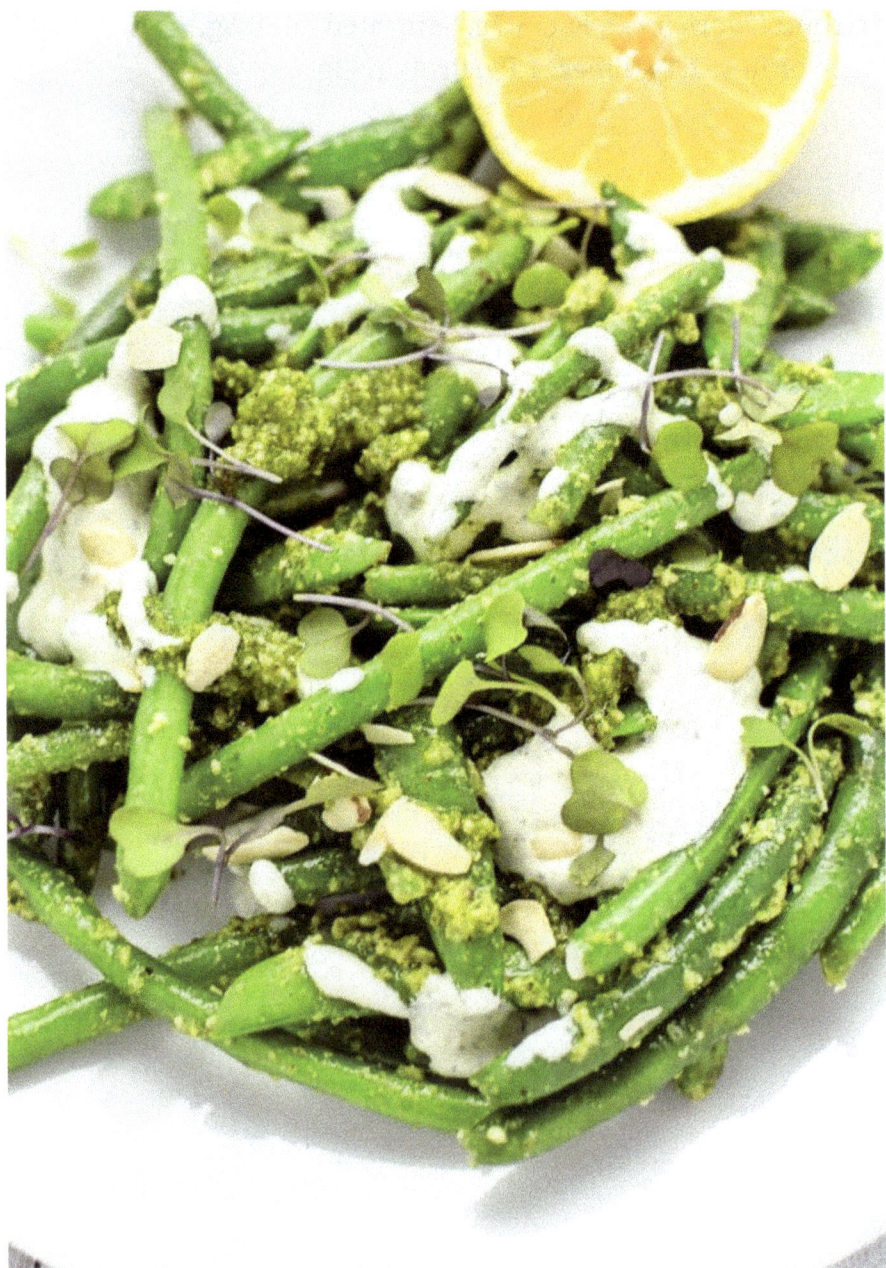

Cucumber Tomato Chopped Salad

Prep Time: 15 minutes

Cook Time: 0 minutes

Serve: 1

Ingredients:

- 1/4 cup light mayonnaise
- 1/2 tablespoon lemon juice
- 1/2 tablespoon fresh dill, chopped
- 1/2 tablespoon chive, chopped
- 1/4 cup feta cheese, crumbled
- Salt and pepper to taste
- 1/2 red onion, chopped
- 1/2 cucumber, diced
- 1/2 radish, diced
- 1 tomato, diced
- Chives, chopped

Instructions:

1.Combine the mayonnaise, lemon juice, fresh dill, chives, feta cheese, salt, and pepper in a bowl.

2.Mix well.

3.Stir in the onion, cucumber, radish, and tomatoes.

4.Coat evenly.

5.Garnish with the chopped chives.

Nutrition: Calories: 187, Fat: 16.7g, Saturated fat: 4.1g, Carbohydrates: 6.7g, Fiber: 2g, Protein: 3.3g

Zucchini Pasta Salad

Prep Time: 4 minutes

Cook Time: 0 minutes

Serve: 1

Ingredients:

- 1 tablespoon olive oil
- 1/2 teaspoons dijon mustard
- 1/3 tablespoons red-wine vinegar
- 1/2 clove garlic, grated
- 2 tablespoons fresh oregano, chopped
- 1/2 shallot, chopped
- ¼ teaspoon red pepper flakes
- 4 oz. zucchini noodles
- ¼ cup Kalamata olives pitted
- 1 cups cherry tomato, sliced in half
- ¾ cup parmesan cheese shaved

Instructions:

1.Mix the olive oil, Dijon mustard, red wine vinegar, garlic, oregano, shallot, and red pepper flakes in a bowl.

2.Stir in the zucchini noodles.

3.Sprinkle on top the olives, tomatoes, and parmesan cheese.

Nutrition: Calories: 299, Fat: 24.7g, Saturated fat: 5.1g, Carbohydrates: 11.6g, Fiber: 2.8g, Protein: 7g

Egg Avocado Salad

Prep Time: 10 minutes

Cook Time: 0 minutes

Serve: 1

Ingredients:

- 1/2 avocado
- 1 hard-boiled egg, peeled and chopped
- 1/4 tablespoon mayonnaise
- 1/4 tablespoons freshly squeezed lemon juice ¼ cup celery, chopped
- 1/2 tablespoons chives, chopped
- Salt and pepper to taste

Instructions:

1.Add the avocado to a large bowl.

2.Mash the avocado using a fork.

3.Stir in the egg and mash the eggs.

4.Add the mayonnaise, lemon juice, celery, chives, salt, and pepper.

5.Chill in the refrigerator for at least 2o to 30 minutes before serving.

Nutrition: Calories: 224, Fat: 18g, Saturated fat: 3.9g, Carbohydrates: 6.1g, Fiber: 3.6g, Protein: 10.6g

Asian Cabbage Salad

Prep Time: 10-15 minutes

Cook Time: 2 minutes

Serve: 4-8

Ingredients:

- 4 C green-cabbage, shredded
- 1/4 C rice wine-vinegar (no sugar added) 1 Tablespoon low sodium soy-sauce
- 4 little spoon Stacey Hawkins Valencia Orange Oil (optional- can be made fat free simply by leaving out)
- 1 normal spoon Asian style seasoning 2 teaspoons lime juice
- 1/4 C cilantro, chopped to taste with salt and pepper

Instructions:

1.Combine shredded cabbage with shredded cabbage in a large bowl, green onions, cilantro, citrus dressing, and Asian seasoning (seeds removed, ground In a coffee grinder, or in a pestle and mortar, with a pestle); mix well. Chill in the refrigerator.

Nutrition: Energy (calories): 99 kcal Protein: 4.13 g Fat: 4.53 g
Carbohydrates: 12.47 g Calcium, Ca92 mg Magnesium, Mg35 mg
Phosphorus, P95 mg

Tangy Kale Salad

Prep Time: 20 minutes

Cook Time: 6 minutes

Serve: 6

Ingredients:

- One-half cup olive oil
- One-fourth cup lemon juice 2 tablespoons Dijon mustard 1 tablespoon minced shallot
- 1 small garlic clove, finely minced
- One-fourth teaspoon salt, or more to taste ground black pepper to taste

Salad:

- 1 teaspoon olive oil
- One-third cup sliced almonds
- 1 bunch kale, center stems discarded and leaves thinly sliced 8 ounces Brussels sprouts, shredded
- 1 cup grated Pecorino Romano cheese

Instructions:

1.Whisk together the lemon Juice to create the dressing, olive oil, shallot, garlic, mustard, ¼ teaspoon salt and pepper. Set aside.

2.To make the salad, heat the oil over medium-high heat in a large skillet. Add the almonds and cook, sometimes stirring, until the almonds are cooked. Almonds are ready. They are fragrant, and the oil is very aromatic about 2 minutes. Transfer to a plate. Attach the skillet to the kale and cook until it begins to wilt and become colorful for about 4 minutes.

3.Add the Brussels sprouts, reduce the heat to medium-low. Season with salt and pepper. Stuff the leaves with the cheese. Drizzle with the dressing.

4.Top with the almonds.

Nutrition: Energy (calories): 193 kcal Protein: 1.74 g Fat: 19.11 g Carbohydrates: 5.56 g Calcium, Ca23 mg Magnesium, Mg14 mg

Crunchy Cauliflower Salad

Prep Time: 10 minutes

Cook Time: 10 minutes

Serve: 8

Ingredients:

- 4 cups cauliflower florets
- 1 Tablespoon (one capful) Stacey Hawkins Tuscan Fantasy Seasoning
- 1/4 cup apple cider vinegar

Instructions:

In a wide bowl,

1.Position the cauliflower florets and coat them with a vinegar solution. Add Stacey Hawkins Tuscan Fantasy Seasoning and stir well. Let sit to allow cauliflower to marinate for 10 minutes.

2.Preheat the oven to 450 degrees and Put a baking sheet on top of it—heavy-duty foil. On a baking sheet, put the marinated cauliflower and bake in the 450-degree oven for 10-12 minutes. Remove and allow to cool.

Nutrition: Energy (calories): 29 kcal Protein: 1.72 g Fat: 0.24 g Carbohydrates: 5.36 g Calcium, Ca20 mg Magnesium, Mg13 mg Phosphorus, P39 mg

Crisp Summer Cucumber Salad

Prep Time: 15 minutes

Cook Time: 0 minutes

Serve: 4

Ingredients:

- 4 C sliced cucumbers (peels on or off- your choice) 2 T apple cider vinegar
- 1/4 C sliced white onion
- 2 tsp Stacey Hawkins Dash of Desperation Seasoning

Instructions:

1. Reserve some cucumber slices for garnish.

2. In a tub, mix up the rest of the ingredients.

3. Pour over remaining cucumber slices and place in a pretty bowl.

4. Enable 15 minutes to sit down to absorb the flavor and serve.

Nutrition: Energy (calories): 20 kcal Protein: 0.29 g Fat: 0.53 g Carbohydrates: 3.08 g Calcium, Ca3 mg Magnesium, Mg3 mg Phosphorus, P6 mg

Mustard Salmon With Herbs

Prep time: 10 min

Cook Time: 30 min

Serving: 2

Ingredients:

- mustard
- mayonnaise
- dressing mix
- garlic powder, or to taste
- lemons
- salmon fillet
- 1 sprig fresh mint, stemmed, or to taste
- 1 sprig fresh rosemary, or to taste
- 2 spoons chopped fresh chives, or to taste
- 1 sprig fresh dill, or to taste
- 4 cloves garlic, crushed, or to taste

Instructions:

1.In a bowl, combine garlic powder, ranch dressing, Italian dressing, mayonnaise, and mustard. Squeeze over the mixture with 1/2 of the lemon. Cut the leftover lemon halves

2.Put the preheated oven in and cook for 30-45 minutes before the flesh can easily flake with a fork.

Nutrition: Calories 277, Fat 11, Carbs 26, Protein 18, Sodium 520

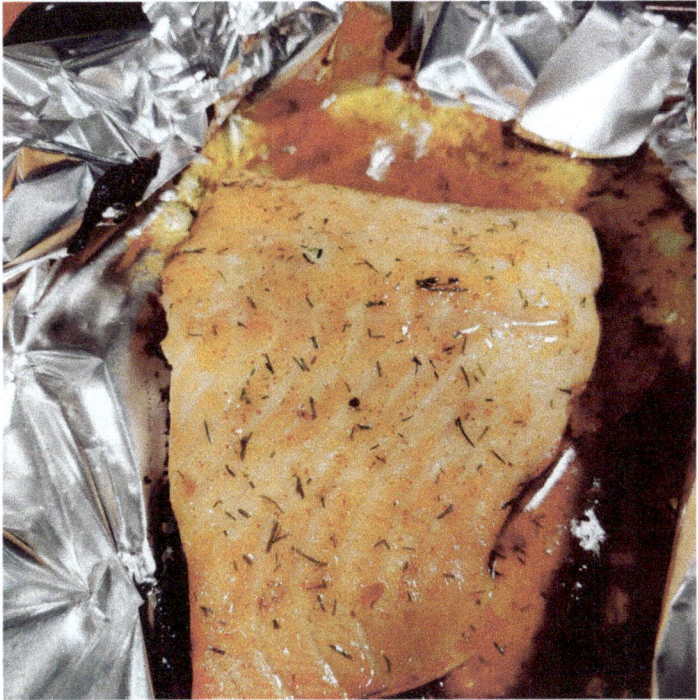

Nutty Coconut Fish

Prep time: 10 min

Cook Time: 30 min

Serving: 2

Ingredients:

- mayonnaise
- mustard
- bread crumbs
- shredded coconut
- mixed nuts
- granulated sugar
- 1 teaspoon salt
- 1/2 teaspoon cayenne pepper
- 1 pound whitefish fillets

Instructions:

1.The oven should be preheated to 190-195 degrees C.

2.Blend brown mustard and mayonnaise in a small bowl. Mix cayenne pepper, salt, sugar, chopped mixed nuts, shredded coconut, and dry breadcrumbs in a medium bowl.

3.Dip fish in mayonnaise mixture, then dip in breadcrumb mixture. In a baking dish, put coated fish fillets.

4.Bake for 20/3 minutes in a preheated oven until the fish flakes easily with a fork.

Nutrition: Calories 180, Fat 2, Carbs 12, Protein 6, Sodium 426

Olive Oil Poached Tuna

Prep time: 10 min

Cook Time: 30 min

Serving: 2

Ingredients:

- tuna steaks
- garlic
- thyme
- pepper flakes
- olive oil
- sea salt to taste

Instructions:

1.Set aside tuna for 10-15 minutes at room temperature.

2.In a heavy pan, mix red pepper flakes, garlic, and thyme. Pour in olive oil until an inch deep. On medium heat, heat for 5-10 minutes until the thyme and garlic sizzles.

3.Put the tuna lightly in the pan of hot oil, then turn heat to low. Cook steaks for 5-7 minutes while constantly spooning oil on top until the tuna is hot and white. Take off heat, move the steaks to a baking pan, and then pour hot oil and herbs on top. Let the fish cool down to temperature.

4.Use plastic wrap to tightly cover the baking dish and put the steaks in the refrigerator for 24 hours. Take the tuna out of the oil and top with sea salt.

Nutrition: Calories 208, Fat 21, Carbs 26, Protein 36, Sodium 543

Tuna Casserole

Prep time: 10 min

Cook Time: 20 min

Serving: 2

Ingredients:

- 1 (16 ounces) package egg noodles
- 1 (10 ounces) package frozen green peas, thawed
- 1/4 cup butter
- 1 (10.75 ounces) can condense cream of mushroom soup
- 1 (5 ounces) can tuna, drained
- 1/4 cup milk
- 1 cup shredded Cheddar cheese

Instructions:

1.Boil a big pot with lightly salted water. Cook pasta in boiling water, till "al dente"; add peas at 3 final minutes of cooking and drain.

2.Melt butter overheats in the same pot. Add Cheddar cheese, milk, tuna, and mushroom soup; mix till mixture is smooth and cheese melts. Mix peas and pasta in till evenly coated.

Nutrition: Calories 398, Fat 16, Carbs 12, Protein 33, Sodium 455

Bacon-Wrapped Salmon

Prep time: 10 min

Cook Time: 30 min

Serving: 2

Ingredients:

- 4 (4 ounces) skin-on salmon fillets
- 1 teaspoon garlic powder
- 1 teaspoon dried dill weed
- salt and pepper to taste
- 1/2 pound bacon, cut in half

Instructions:

1.Preheat oven to 375°F. Generously brush olive oil on a cookie sheet.

2.Arrange salmon fillets skin down on the cookie sheet. Season fillets with dill, salt, pepper, and garlic powder. Cover the fillets completely with bacon strips. Arrange the bacon so they don't overlap each other.

3.Bake in the oven for 20-23 minutes, just until the fish's center is not translucent. To broil, change the oven setting and cook for another 1 to 2 minutes until the bacon becomes crispy.

Nutrition: Calories 307, Fat 23, Carbs 8, Protein 16, Sodium 590

Bagna Cauda

Prep time: 10 min

Cook Time: 30 min

Serving: 2

Ingredients:

- 1/2 cup butter
- 10 cloves garlic, minced
- fillets
- cream

Instructions:

1.Mix in garlic and cook until softened. Lower the heat to low. Mix in heavy cream and anchovy filets.

2.Bring the mixture back to medium heat, stirring from time to time, until bubbling. Serve hot.

Nutrition: Calories 670, Fat 34, Carbs 26, Protein 28, Sodium 430

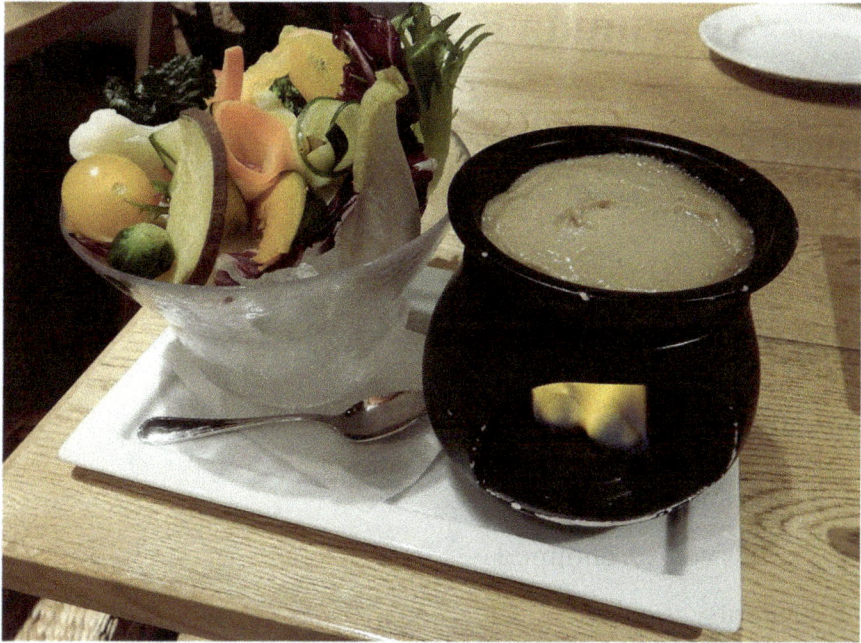

Bermuda Fish Chowder

Prep time: 10 min

Cook Time: 30 min

Serving: 2

Ingredients:

- 2 tablespoons vegetable oil
- 3 stalks celery, chopped
- 2 carrots, chopped
- 1 onion, chopped
- 1 green bell pepper, chopped
- 3 cloves garlic, minced
- 3 tablespoons tomato paste
- 4 cups clam juice
- 2 potatoes, peeled and cubed
- 1 (14.5 ounces) can peeled tomatoes
- 2 spoons Worcestershire sauce
- 1 jalapeno pepper
- 1 little spoon ground black pepper
- 1 bay-leaf
- 1 pound red-snapper fillets, cut into 1 inch pieces

Instructions:

1.In a large soup pot, heat the oil over medium heat. Toss in the carrots, celery, green pepper, onion, and garlic and sauté them for about 8 minutes.

2.Pour in the tomato paste and cook and stir for 1 minute. Mix in the clam juice, canned tomatoes with juice, potatoes, Worcestershire sauce, bay leaf, jalapeno pepper, and ground black pepper. Let it simmer until the potatoes are already tender, stirring the soup for about every 30 minutes.

3.Put the fish in and let it simmer for about 10 minutes until the snapper easily flakes with a fork.

Nutrition: Calories 320, Fat 28, Carbs 21, Protein 36, Sodium 660

Salmon Tikka

Prep time: 10 min

Cook Time: 30 min

Serving: 2

Ingredients:

- red pepper
- turmeric
- salt
- salmon fillets
- cornstarch
- oil

Instructions:

1.In a bowl, combine salt, turmeric, and cayenne. Put salmon into the bowl; toss until evenly coated with seasoning mixture. Let fish rest for 15 minutes.

2.In a container, heat oil over medium heat. Meanwhile, sprinkle cornstarch all over salmon; toss to coat evenly.

3.Cook salmon in hot oil, about 1 minute on each side, until golden brown.

Nutrition: Calories 254, Fat 24, Carbs 12, Protein 26, Sodium 765

Almond And Parmesan Crusted Tilapia

Prep time: 10 min

Cook Time: 30 min

Serving: 2

Ingredients:

- 1 teaspoon olive oil, or as needed
- 3 cloves garlic, minced
- 1/2 cup grated Parmesan cheese
- almonds, crushed
- mayonnaise
- bread crumbs
- 2 tablespoons fresh lemon juice
- 1/4 teaspoon dried basil
- 1/4 teaspoon ground black pepper
- 1/8 teaspoon onion powder
- 1/8 teaspoon celery salt
- 1 pound tilapia fillets

Instructions:

1.Put the rack 6 inches away from the heat source and start preheating the oven's broiler. Use aluminum foil to line a broiling tray or use olive oil cooking spray to coat.

2.Heat olive oil in a frying container over medium heat, stir garlic while cooking for 3 to 5 minutes, or aromatic.

3.In a bowl, combine celery salt, onion powder, black pepper, basil, seafood seasoning, lemon juice, bread crumbs, mayonnaise, almonds, buttery spreads, garlic, and Parmesan cheese.

4.Set the tilapia fillets in a layer on top of the prepared pan, use aluminum foil to cover it.

5.Put the container in the preheated oven and start boiling for about 2 to 3 minutes. Flip the fillets, cover the pan with aluminum foil, and restart broiling for 2 to 3 more minutes. Remove aluminum foil and put the Parmesan cheese mixture on top to cover the fish. Broil in the oven for 2 more minutes until topping gets browned; fish can be shredded easily with a fork.

Nutrition: Calories 498, Fat 32, Carbs 26, Protein 8, Sodium 634

Crab And Shrimp Pasta Salad

Prep time: 10 min

Cook Time: 30 min

Serving: 2

Ingredients:

- 1 (16 ounces) package uncooked tri-colored spiral pasta
- 1/2 cup mayonnaise
- 1/4 cup apple cider vinegar
- 1/4 cup olive oil
- salt and pepper to taste
- 1 (8 ounces) package imitation crabmeat, flaked
- 1 (6.5 ounces) can tiny shrimp, drained
- 1-pint grape tomatoes halved
- 1 English cucumber, diced
- 1 (4 ounces) can slice black olives, drained
- 1 red bell pepper, seeded and chopped

Instructions:

1.Boil a big pot with lightly salted water. Add pasta. Cook for 10 minutes till tender, then drain. Cool by rinsing under cold water. Put into a big bowl, put aside.

2.Mix pepper, salt, olive oil, vinegar, and mayonnaise in a small bowl. Put on pasta; mix to coat. Add bell pepper, black olives, cucumber, tomatoes, shrimp, and crab. Gently mix to coat in dressing. Taste, then adjust seasoning if you want. Mix extra mayonnaise if the pasta is very dry.

Nutrition: Calories 480, Fat 24, Carbs 10, Protein 23, Sodium 680

Cream Of Salmon Soup

Prep time: 10 min

Cook Time: 30 min

Serving: 2

Ingredients:

Puff Pastry Triangles:

- 1 sheet frozen puff pastry, thawed
- 1 egg yolk, beaten
- 1 tablespoon sesame seeds

Salmon Soup:

- 1 1/2 tablespoons butter
- 1 onion, diced
- 18 ounces salmon fillets, diced
- 1 tablespoon tomato paste
- 2 1/2 cups fish stock
- 1/2 cup dry white wine
- 1 tablespoon cornstarch
- 1 1/4 cups heavy whipping cream
- A little saffron, salt and white pepper, freshly ground, to taste

- 3 little spoons chopped fresh dill

Instructions:

1.Set the oven at 400°F and start preheating.

2.On a lightly floured surface, place puff pastry; use a rolling pin to roll it out. Brush egg yolk over. Put sesame seeds on top; press in firmly. First, divide puff pastry into squares, then into triangles, put them on a baking sheet.

3.Start baking for about 15 minutes in the preheated oven till triangles are puffed up and golden brown.

4.In the meantime, place a pot on medium heat, melt in the butter and cook in onion till soft and translucent, about 5 minutes. 5.Include in salmon and cook for 5 minutes. Mix in tomato paste; cook for 1 minute. Add in white wine and fish stock. Boil everything; turn down the heat; simmer for 15 minutes. Let it boil.

6.Blend a little bit of water and cornstarch into a paste. Pour into the soup and let the mixture come to a boil. Cook till the soup is thickened, about 5 minutes. Make the soup into a smooth purée with an immersion blender. Mix in saffron and cream. Flavor with pepper and salt.

7.Dill for garnish and puff pastry triangles to serve with the soup.

Nutrition: Calories 436, Fat 32, Carbs 26, Protein 36, Sodium 663

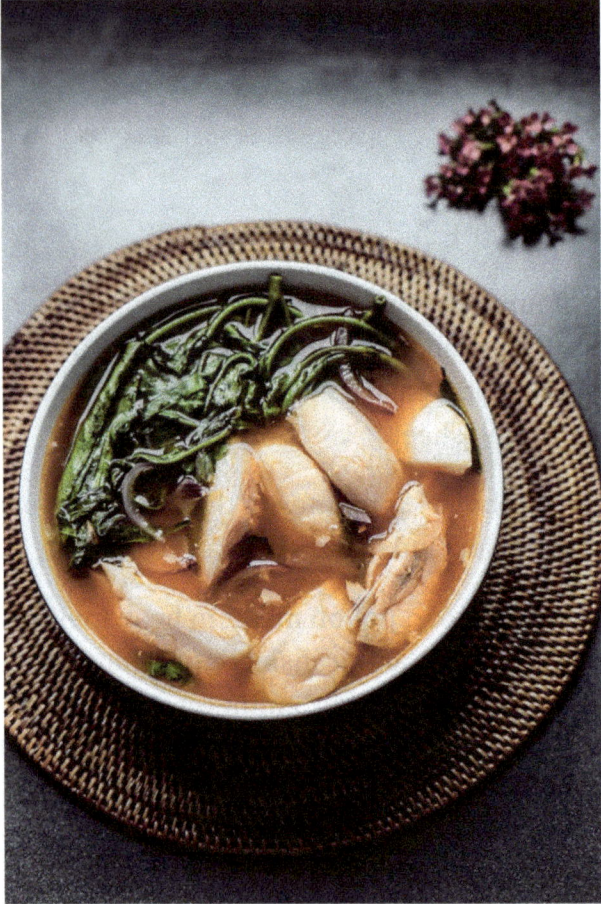

Creamed Salmon On Toast

Prep time: 10 min

Cook Time: 30 min

Serving: 2

Ingredients:

- Butter
- flour
- milk
- green peas
- 1 (14.75 ounces) can salmon
- salt and pepper to taste

Instructions:

1.Set the heat to medium, then melt butter in a skillet or saucepan. Whisk the flour while stirring continuously to have a smooth paste. Carefully pour the milk while stirring continuously with the peas' leftover liquids to make a smooth thick gravy.

2.Break large pieces of the salmon into smaller pieces by flaking them into a bowl. Mix the peas and salmon carefully into the sauce using a wooden spoon to keep the peas from being mashed. Cook until thoroughly heated.

3.Use a toaster oven or a broiler pan to toast some bread. You can even add butter if you want and garnish it with some salmon mixture on top.

Nutrition: Calories 244, Fat 32, Carbs 26, Protein 6, Sodium 321

Coconut Salsa on Chipotle Fish Tacos

Prep Time: 10 minutes

Cook Time: 10 minutes

Serve: 4

Ingredients:

- ¼ cup chopped fresh cilantro
- ½ cup seeded and finely chopped plum tomato
- 1 cup peeled and finely chopped mango
- 1 lime cut into wedges
- 1 tablespoon chipotle Chile powder
- 1 tablespoon safflower oil
- 1/3 cup finely chopped red onion
- 10 tablespoon fresh lime juice, divided
- 4 6-oz boneless, skinless cod fillets
- 5 tablespoon dried unsweetened shredded coconut
- 8 pcs of 6-inch tortillas, heated

Instructions:

1. Whisk well Chile powder, oil, and 4 tablespoon lime juice in a glass baking dish. Add cod and marinate for 12 – 15 minutes. Turning once halfway through the marinating time.

2. Make the salsa by mixing coconut, 6 tablespoon lime juice, cilantro, onions, tomatoes and mangoes in a medium bowl. Set aside.

3. On high, heat a grill pan. Place cod and grill for four minutes per side, turning only once.

4. Once cooked, slice cod into large flakes and evenly divide onto the tortilla.

5. Evenly divide salsa on top of cod and serve with a side of lime wedges.

Nutrition: Calories: 477 Protein: 35.0g Fat: 12.4g Carbs: 57.4g

Baked Cod Crusted with Herbs

Prep Time: 5 minutes

Cook Time: 10 minutes

Serve: 4

Ingredients:

- ¼ cup honey
- ¼ teaspoon salt
- ½ cup panko
- ½ teaspoon pepper
- 1 tablespoon extra virgin olive oil
- 1 tablespoon lemon juice
- 1 teaspoon dried basil
- 1 teaspoon dried parsley
- 1 teaspoon rosemary
- 4 pieces of 4-oz cod fillets

Instructions:

1. With olive oil, grease a 9 x 13-inch baking pan and preheat oven to 375oF.

2. In a zip-top bag, mix panko, rosemary, salt, pepper, parsley and basil.

3. Evenly spread cod fillets in a prepped dish and drizzle with lemon juice.

4. Then brush the fillets with honey on all sides. Discard remaining honey, if any.

5. Then evenly divide the panko mixture on top of cod fillets.

6. Pop in the oven and bake for ten minutes or until fish is cooked.

Nutrition: Calories: 137 Protein: 5g Fat: 2g Carbs: 21g

Cajun Garlic Shrimp Noodle Bowl

Prep Time: 10 minutes

Cook Time: 15 minutes

Serve: 2

Ingredients:

- ½ teaspoon salt
- 1 onion, sliced
- 1 red pepper, sliced
- 1 tablespoon butter
- 1 teaspoon garlic granules
- 1 teaspoon onion powder
- 1 teaspoon paprika
- 2 large zucchinis, cut into noodle strips
- 20 jumbo shrimps, shells removed and deveined
- 3 cloves garlic, minced
- 3 tablespoon ghee
- A dash of cayenne pepper
- A dash of red pepper flakes

Instructions:

1. Prepare the Cajun seasoning by mixing the onion powder, garlic granules, pepper flakes, cayenne pepper, paprika and salt. Toss in the shrimp to coat in the seasoning.

2. In a skillet, heat the ghee and sauté the garlic. Add in the red pepper and onions and continue sautéing for 4 minutes.

3. Add the Cajun shrimp and cook until opaque. Set aside.

4. In another pan, heat the butter and sauté the zucchini noodles for three minutes.

5. Assemble by placing the Cajun shrimps on top of the zucchini noodles.

Nutrition: Calories: 712 Fat: 30.0g Protein: 97.8g Carbs: 20.2g

Saganaki Shrimp

Prep Time: 10 minutes

Cook Time: 10 minutes

Serve: 4

Ingredients:

- ¼ teaspoon salt
- ½ cup Chardonnay
- ½ cup crumbled Greek feta cheese
- 1 medium bulb. fennel, cored and finely chopped
- 1 small Chile pepper, seeded and minced
- 1 tablespoon extra virgin olive oil
- 12 jumbo shrimps, deveined with tails left on
- 2 tablespoon lemon juice, divided
- 5 scallions sliced thinly
- Pepper to taste

Instructions:

1. In a medium bowl, mix salt, lemon juice and shrimp.

2. On medium fire, place a saganaki pan (or large nonstick saucepan) and heat oil.

3. Sauté Chile pepper, scallions, and fennel for 4 minutes or until starting to brown and is already soft.

4. Add wine and sauté for another minute.

5. Place shrimps on top of the fennel, cover and cook for 4 minutes or until shrimps are pink.

6. Remove just the shrimp and transfer to a plate.

7. Add pepper, feta and 1 tablespoon lemon juice to the pan and cook for a minute or until cheese begins to melt.

8. To serve, place cheese and fennel mixture on a serving plate and top with shrimps.

Nutrition: Calories: 310 Protein: 49.7g Fat: 6.8g Carbs: 8.4g

Creamy Bacon-Fish Chowder

Prep Time: 10 minutes

Cook Time: 30 minutes

Serve: 8

Ingredients:

- 1 1/2 lbs. cod
- 1 1/2 teaspoon dried thyme
- 1 large onion, chopped
- 1 medium carrot, coarsely chopped
- 1 tablespoon butter, cut into small pieces
- 1 teaspoon salt, divided
- 3 1/2 cups baking potato, peeled and cubed
- 3 slices uncooked bacon
- 3/4 teaspoon ground black pepper, divided
- 4 1/2 cups water
- 4 bay leaves
- 4 cups 2% reduced-fat milk

Instructions:

1. In a large skillet, add the water and bay leaves and let it simmer. Add the fish. Cover and let it simmer some more until the flesh

flakes easily with a fork. Remove the fish from the skillet and cut it into large pieces. Set aside the cooking liquid.

2. Place Dutch oven in medium heat and cook the bacon until crisp. Remove the bacon and reserve the bacon drippings. Crush the bacon and set aside.

3. Stir potato, onion and carrot in the pan with the bacon drippings, cook over medium heat for 10 minutes. Add the cooking liquid, bay leaves, 1/2 teaspoon salt, 1/4 teaspoon pepper and thyme, let it boil. Lower the heat and let simmer for 11 minutes. Add the milk and butter, simmer until the potatoes become tender, but do not boil. Add the fish, 1/2 teaspoon salt, 1/2 teaspoon pepper. Remove the bay leaves.

4. Serve sprinkled with the crushed bacon.

Nutrition: Calories: 400 Carbs: 34.5g Protein: 20.8g Fat: 19.7g

Crisped Coco-Shrimp with Mango Dip

Prep Time: 10 minutes

Cook Time: 20 minutes

Serve: 4

Ingredients:

- 1 cup shredded coconut
- 1 lb. raw shrimp, peeled and deveined
- 2 egg whites
- 4 tablespoon tapioca starch
- Pepper and salt to tast
- Mango Dip Ingredients:
- 1 cup mango, chopped
- 1 jalapeño, thinly minced
- 1 teaspoon lime juice
- 1/3 cup coconut milk
- 3 teaspoon raw honey

Instructions:

1. preheat oven to 400oF.

2. Ready a pan with a wire rack on top.

3. In a medium bowl, add tapioca starch and season with pepper and salt.

4. In a second medium bowl, add egg whites and whisk.

5. In a third medium bowl, add coconut.

6. To ready shrimps, dip first in tapioca starch, then egg whites, and then coconut. Place dredged shrimp on wire rack. Repeat until all shrimps are covered.

7. Pop shrimps in the oven and roast for 10 minutes per side.

8. Meanwhile, make the dip by adding all ingredients in a blender. Puree until smooth and creamy. Transfer to a dipping bowl.

9. Once shrimps are golden brown, serve with mango dip.

Nutrition: Calories: 294.2 Protein: 26.6g Fat: 7g Carbs: 31.2g

Cucumber-Basil Salsa on Halibut Pouches

Prep Time: 10 minutes

Cook Time: 17 minutes

Serve: 4

Ingredients:

- 1 lime, thinly sliced into eight pieces
- 2 cups mustard greens, stems removed
- 2 teaspoon olive oil
- 4 – 5 radishes trimmed and quartered
- 4 4-oz skinless halibut filets
- 4 large fresh basil leaves
- Cayenne pepper to taste – optional
- Pepper and salt to taste
- Salsa Ingredients:
- 1 ½ cups diced cucumber
- 1 ½ finely chopped fresh basil leaves
- 2 teaspoon fresh lime juice
- Pepper and salt to taste

Instructions:

1. preheat oven to 400°F.

2. Prepare parchment papers by making 4 pieces of 15 x 12-inch rectangles. Lengthwise, fold in half and unfold pieces on the table.

3. Season halibut fillets with pepper, salt and cayenne—if using cayenne.

4. Just to the right of the fold, place ½ cup of mustard greens. Add a basil leaf on the center of mustard greens and topped with 1 lime slice. Around the greens, layer ¼ of the radishes. Drizzle with ½ teaspoon of oil, season with pepper and salt. Top it with a slice of halibut fillet.

5. Just as you would make a calzone, fold the parchment paper over your filling and crimp the edges of the parchment paper beginning from one end to the other end. To seal the end of the crimped parchment paper, pinch it.

6. Repeat the remaining ingredients until you have 4 pieces of parchment papers filled with halibut and greens.

7. Place pouches in a pan and bake in the oven until halibut is flaky around 15 to 17 minutes.

8. While waiting for halibut pouches to cook, make your salsa by mixing all salsa ingredients in a medium bowl.

9. Once halibut is cooked, remove it from the oven and make a tear on top. Be careful of the steam as it is very hot. Equally, divide salsa and spoon ¼ of salsa on top of halibut through the slit you have created.

Nutrition: Calories: 335.4 Protein: 20.2g Fat: 16.3g Carbs: 22.1g

Salmon with Mustard

Prep Time: 10 minutes

Cook Time: 8 minutes

Serve: 4

Ingredients:

- ¼ teaspoon ground red pepper or chili powder
- ¼ teaspoon ground turmeric
- ¼ teaspoon salt
- 1 teaspoon honey
- 1/8 teaspoon garlic powder or a minced clove garlic 2 teaspoon. whole grain mustard 4 pcs 6-oz salmon fillets

Instructions:

1. In a small bowl, mix well salt, garlic powder, red pepper, turmeric, honey and mustard.

2. Preheat the oven to broil and grease a baking dish with cooking spray.

3. Place salmon on a baking dish with skin side down and spread evenly mustard mixture on top of salmon.

4. Pop in the oven and broil until flaky, around 8 minutes.

Nutrition: Calories: 324 Fat: 18.9 g Protein: 34 g Carbs: 2.9g

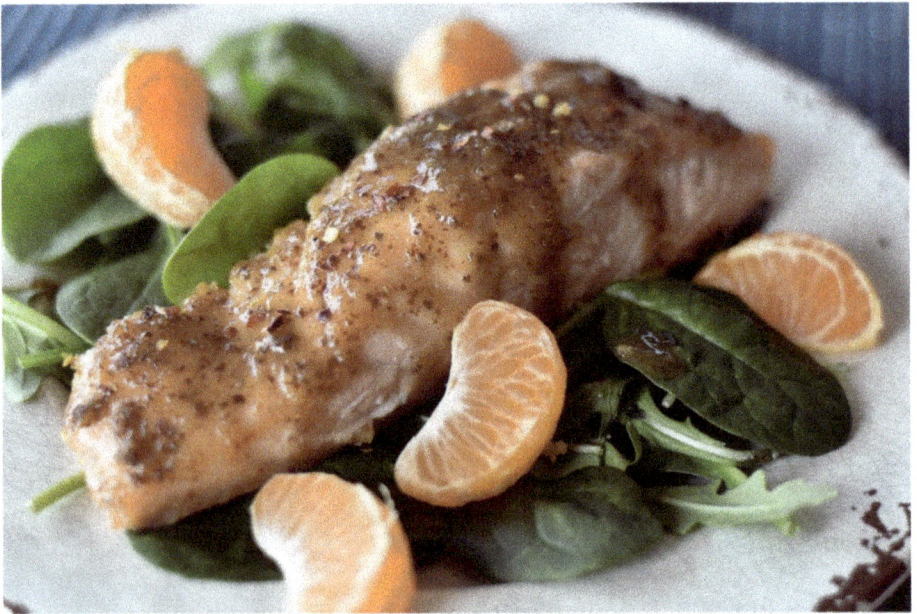

Dijon Mustard and Lime Marinated Shrimp

Prep Time: 10 minutes

Cook Time: 10 minutes

Serve: 8

Ingredients:

- ½ cup fresh lime juice and lime zest as garnish
- ½ cup of rice vinegar
- ½ teaspoon hot sauce
- 1 bay leaf
- 1 cup of water
- 1 lb. uncooked shrimp, peeled and deveined
- 1 medium red onion, chopped
- 2 tablespoon capers
- 2 tablespoon Dijon mustard
- 3 whole cloves

Instructions:

1. Mix hot sauce, mustard, capers, lime juice and onion in a shallow baking dish and set aside.

2. Put the bay leaf, cloves, vinegar, and water to a boil in a large saucepan.

3. Once boiling, add shrimps and cook for a minute while stirring continuously.

4. Drain shrimps and pour shrimps into onion mixture.

5. For an hour, refrigerate while covered the shrimps.

6. Then serve shrimps cold and garnished with lime zest.

Nutrition: Calories: 232.2 Protein: 17.8g Fat: 3g Carbs: 15g

Dill Relish on White Sea Bass

Prep Time: 10 minutes

Cook Time: 12 minutes

Serve: 4

Ingredients:

- 1 ½ tablespoon chopped white onion
- 1 ½ teaspoon chopped fresh dill
- 1 lemon, quartered
- 1 teaspoon Dijon mustard
- 1 teaspoon lemon juice
- 1 teaspoon pickled baby capers, drained
- 4 pieces of 4-oz white sea bass fillets

Instructions:

1. Preheat oven to 375°F.

2. Mix lemon juice, mustard, dill, capers and onions in a small bowl.

3. Prepare four aluminum foil squares and place 1 fillet per foil.

4. Squeeze a lemon wedge per fish.

5. Evenly divide into 4 the dill spread and drizzle over the fillet.

6. Close the foil over the fish securely and pop in the oven.

7. Bake for 12 minutes or until fish is cooked through.

8. Remove from foil and transfer to a serving platter.

Nutrition: Calories: 115 Protein: 7g Fat: 1g Carbs: 12g

Salmon & Arugula Omelet

Prep Time: 10 minutes

Cook Time: 7 minutes

Serve: 4

Ingredients:

- 6 eggs
- 2 tablespoons unsweetened almond milk Salt and ground black pepper, as required 2 tablespoons olive oil
- 4 ounces smoked salmon, cut into bite-sized chunks
- 2 cups fresh arugula, chopped finely
- 4 scallions, chopped finely

Instructions:

1.In a bowl, place the eggs, coconut milk, salt and black pepper and beat well. Set aside.

2. Over medium pressure, heat the oil in a non-stick skillet.

3.Place the egg mixture evenly and cook for about 30 seconds without stirring.

4.Place the salmon kale and scallions on top of egg mixture evenly.

5. Lower the heat to a low level and cook covered for about 4-5 minutes or until omelet is done completely.

6.Uncover the skillet and cook for about 1 minute.

7.Carefully transfer the omelet onto a serving plate.

Tuna Omelet

Prep Time: 10 minutes

Cook Time: 5 minutes

Serve: 2

Ingredients:

- 4 eggs
- ¼ cup unsweetened almond milk
- 1 tablespoon scallions, chopped
- 1 garlic clove, minced
- ½ of jalapeño pepper, minced
- Salt and ground black pepper, to taste
- 1 (5-ounce) can water-packed tuna, drained and flaked
- 1 tablespoon olive oil
- 3 normal spoons green bell pepper, seeded and chopped
- 3 tablespoons tomato, chopped
- ¼ cup low-fat cheddar cheese, shredded

Instructions:

1. In a bowl, add the eggs, almond milk, scallions, garlic, jalapeño pepper, salt, and black pepper, and beat well.

2. Add the tuna and stir to combine.

3.In a big-non-stick frying pan, heat oil over medium heat.

4.Place the egg mixture in an even layer and cook for about 1–2 minutes, without stirring.

5.Carefully lift the edges to run the uncooked portion flow underneath.

6.Spread the veggies over the egg mixture and sprinkle with the cheese.

7.Cover the frying pan and cook for about 30–60 seconds.

8.Remove the lid and fold the omelet in half.

9.Remove from the heat and cut the omelet into 2 portions.

Fish Stew

Prep Time: 15 minutes

Cook Time: 50 minutes

Serve: 10

Ingredients:

- ¼ cup coconut oil
- ½ cup yellow onion, chopped
- 1 cup celery stalk, chopped
- ½ cup green bell pepper, seeded and chopped
- 1 garlic clove, minced
- 4 cups water
- 4 beef bouillon cubes
- 20 ounces okra, trimmed and chopped
- 2 (14-ounce) cans sugar-free diced tomatoes with liquid
- 2 bay leaves
- 1 teaspoon dried thyme, crushed
- 2 teaspoons red pepper flakes, crushed
- ¼ teaspoon hot pepper sauce
- Salt and ground black pepper, as required
- 32 ounces catfish fillets
- ½ cup fresh cilantro, chopped

Instructions:

1.In a big skillet, melt the coconut oil over medium heat and sauté the onion, celery and bell pepper for about 4-5 minutes.

2.Meanwhile, in a large soup pan, mix together bouillon cubes and water and bring to a boil over medium heat.

3.Transfer the onion mixture and remaining ingredients except catfish into the pan of boiling water and bring to a boil.

4.Decrease the heat to low, cook for about 30 minutes, protected.

5.Stir in catfish fillets and cook for about 10-15 minutes.

6. Stir in the cilantro and remove from the heat.

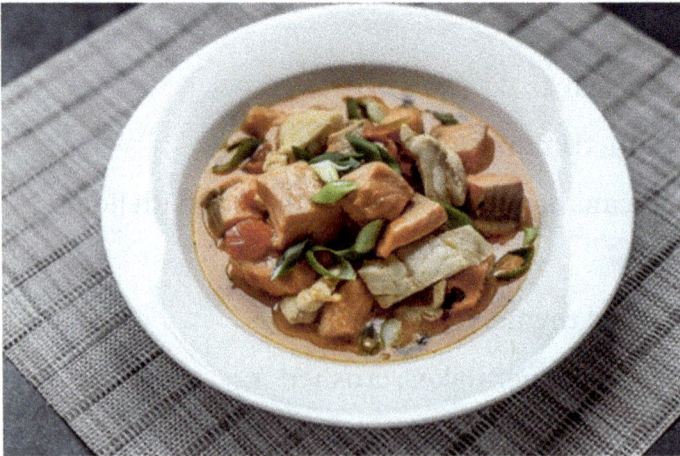

www.ingramcontent.com/pod-product-compliance
Lightning Source LLC
Chambersburg PA
CBHW050748030426
42336CB00012B/1709